WHY ME WANT EAT

WANT EAT

FIXING YOUR FOOD
F*CKEDUPITUDE

Krista Scott-Dixon, PhD

Are you lost?

Good, then let's go exploring together...

Disclaimer:
This is not your average
self-help book.

You might have noticed some swears already. Like in the title. There will be lots more of those.

I'm going to call a shit a shit.

If gentler language or lots of Oprah hugs is more your style, I suggest you put this book down immediately, and go recover with an ice pack and some chamomile tea.

No hard feelings. No judgement.

I'm a coach, not a shrink.

I highly recommend you also go get some therapy from an actual therapist. That stuff is the shizznit. Seriously.

My experience is my experience.

It probably won't be just like yours.

At the same time, we probably share some stuff that might help you to know.

Take what you can use, and leave the rest.

Find the nuggets that work for you.

Despite the title, this book won't fix you.

But it's a damn good start. At least I think so.

Here we go.

Read this book any way you like.

Do anything you like after reading it.

Go as fast or as slowly as you like.

Read it out loud, or quietly, or one word at a time, or scan it all at once.

Start at the beginning.

Or start at the end.

Or randomly pick a page.

It's your show. There are no rules.

YOU are in control of your experience here.

Hello.

I'm Krista. People call me KSD though.

I like cursing. A lot.

I once felt pretty fucked up. And now I don't.

I felt fucked up about a lot of things.

One of those things was food and eating and exercise and body stuff. (Technically I guess that's four things. I haven't fixed being fucked up at math yet.)

Being fucked up is sometimes fun. (More on this later.)

But most of the time, feeling fucked up kinda sucks. Or really sucks.

If you've picked up this book, you may be feeling fucked up too.

Maybe that doesn't feel great to you either.

Maybe you're not even sure you want to change right now.

That's OK.

You do you. Your path is your path.

There's no right way to be, or feel, or do things.

Take your time.

It may feel super urgent that you *fix everything right now!!!!*

Especially if you're just sick and tired of being sick and tired and you want to get off whatever crazy train you're on.

I get that.

Go fast, if you prefer.

At the same time:

There is no rush.

You can look at this book forever if you want.

Doing nothing is always an option.

(Or, as the Zen folks say, "When nothing works, do nothing.")

I'm just going to give you some suggestions and some swears.

You decide what works for you.

Deal?

Just enough about me not to bore the shit out of you...

If you ever want to know how a helping professional is fucked up, look at what their specialty is.

Marriage counsellors have often had shit relationships. Physical therapists have often had injuries. Addictions counsellors probably woke up in a dumpster one day and decided enough was enough.

I work in the field of health, fitness, and nutrition.

So guess how I was fucked up?!

Of course — about food, eating and not-eating, exercise, and body image.

When I was first fucked up, I got really confused.

I didn't "fit the profile" of a good little eating disorder.

I was older. (My shit started in my mid-30s.)

I was not the product of crappy parenting, besides being subjected to epic dad humour.

I didn't want to be *skinny*. I wanted to be *riptshizzled* — strong, lean, jacked, fearsome.

I didn't do stuff like barf on purpose. I can't even barf on purpose when I've eaten bad shrimp salad and desperately want to.

I told myself I was "being healthy". Healthy people don't get fucked up, right?

I didn't make sense, even to myself.

So it took me a long time to realize that I was doing a thing called "disordered eating". I was alternating starving with binge eating, and having lots of weird food hangups.

Plus "compensating", with tons of exercise.

Plus having "body dysmorphia". Which means a lot of poking and pinching and weighing and looking in the mirror and being sad and anxious and self-critical and ashamed.

Plus being "perfectionist", which I always thought was about being perfect but in reality is more about having rigid and dysfunctional ways of thinking like *If there's a tiny mistake then things are fucked* or *Everyone is judging me and boy am I failing here* or *I've already screwed up so I might as well keep going and screw up some more.*

And keep going I did.

Someone told me, "You look like you got out of a prison camp." I kept going.

I lost my period and basically stopped making all hormones altogether. I kept going.

I sometimes ate so much I could barely

breathe. I kept going.

Because achievement! Dare to dream! Be awesome! No excuses! Other people are judging! Look at this muffin top I still have!

And so forth.

When I was lying in the cranial MRI that was measuring whether I had a pituitary tumour that might explain why my shit was so wack, I had a lot of time to think.

I decided I didn't want to be menopausal at 35 because my body thought I might be dying.

I didn't want food and eating and not-eating and exercise and my neuroses to be the only thing I thought and talked about.

I didn't want to be sad and anxious and crazy and weird and obsessed and hurting.

I wanted to be happy and healthy and secure and loving other people and myself. And just not so fucking whackadoodle crazy all the damn time.

So:

I chose to change.

And so can you.

No matter where you are in your journey.

You are probably going to feel things when you read this.

Maybe you'll feel mad, or sad, or numb, or anxious, or defensive, or screamy. Or something else that you can't even name.

Maybe you'll be pissed at me, pissed at your parents, pissed at schoolyard bullies, pissed at the world, pissed at everything. Rarrrr!!!

Maybe this book will bring up some grody shit for you.

Like some hardcore, gnarly, scummy stuff — imagine a ball of dryer lint mixed with old chewing gum mixed with dog poo that you just fished out of your shower drain kind of scummy stuff.

Be safe. Be kind. Take care of yourself.

Love yourself as much as you can right now.

Reach out for help and support from folks you trust. If you don't have those folks, start looking, because we all need them.

Any feeling is valid.

Just because this book might make you feel bad, doesn't mean *it's* wrong… or that *you're* wrong.

Just let the feelz tap dance as they choose, and try to stay calm.

As much as you can, stay aware of what you are feeling, sensing, and thinking.

As you read, pause as you need to.

Digest.

Take breaks and check in.

What's happening?

What is this?

What am I noticing?

Whatever it is, it's all normal.

Simply observe it.

Pay attention.

Get what's in your head out of it.

If ideas, or thoughts, or feelings, or other things come up, capture them.

Grab a pen and start scribbling in the margins, or in a notebook.

Crumple up what you write, if you like, and whip it across the room while yelling "FUCK YOU!" Stomp on it.

Or print each letter out in beautiful cursive, with a sparkly scented marker, or a ridiculously expensive fountain pen, and then illuminate it lovingly like a medieval manuscript.

Or doodle. Or finger paint. Or make crafts out of googly eyes, pasta shells, and cotton balls.

Or do an interpretive dance. Or invent new farm animal noises like *squeeeaaagghh-ooka-ooka*.

Whatever works for you. Just express yourself.

Get stuff out of your brain and into the world.

You can share this stuff. Or keep it just for you. Your own private space.

Even if nobody else ever sees it, getting stuff out of your head can transform it, often in magical and unanticipated ways.

Try capturing something.

Write down what you're thinking or feeling right now.

_____

_____

_____

_____

_____

_____

OR, DOODLE WHAt YOU'RE tHINKING OR FEELING RIGHt NOW.

STICK SOME GOOGLY EYES HERE.

Observe what you're feeling in your body, if you can.

Lots of us get into eating and food weirdness because we're trying to avoid feeling anything, especially the bad stuff.

Even a quick scan of your physical sensations can tell you a lot, and help keep you grounded.

You don't have to feel or notice *everything* right now.

Just try noticing *a little bit*.

Start with noticing just your elbow. Or your ankle. Or your right eye.

Or what your tongue is doing in your mouth.

Body sensations are like your car's dashboard indicator lights.

They give you important — maybe even essential — information.

More on this later.

Try a quick scan of your body now. What do you notice?

Circle any word that seems to fit.

hot	alert	confined
cold	achey	fidgety
itchy	crampy	lethargic
heavy	jumpy	energetic
light	spacey	open
pain	breathless	squished
restless	tingly	dizzy
relaxed	tight	suffocated
tense	loose	sweaty
calm	yucky	bubbly
congested	bloated	jaw-grinding
clear	sniffly	burny
tired	burpy	soft
awake	groovy	hard
nauseated	bruised	flowing
blah	restricted	warmth

Other stuff you notice:

_____

_____

_____

_____

_____

OR, DOODLE A PICTURE OF
HOW YOUR BODY FEELS RIGHt
NOW.

What's your story?

Why did you start reading this book?

Do you feel fucked up about food, or eating, or not-eating, or exercise, or body stuff?

Do you think you *might* be fucked up, but aren't sure? (Or don't want to be sure?)

Do you just feel like things could be better, somehow?

Do you feel perfectly fine, and you're just curious?

Do you know someone else who's fucked up and want to help them?

Are you stuck in a waiting room and just bored, and this beats old copies of *Reader's Digest*?

There's no right or wrong reason for being here.

Maybe you don't know all the reasons why. Maybe you'll never know.

That's OK.

For now, try making a list of what you hope to get out of this book.

Write down what you hope to get out of this book.

_____

_____

_____

_____

_____

_____

_____

OR, DOODLE A PICTURE OF
WHAT YOU HOPE to GET OUT
OF tHIS BOOK.

MAKE A SCRIBBLE HERE.
SEE IF YOU CAN StAB tHE PEN
RIGHt tHROUGH tHE PAPER.

(Almost) all of us are fucked up.

I say "almost", because humans are terrible at fitting into neat little boxes. There's always That Person who messes up the data.

In this case, there's probably someone — probably a few someones — out there who are perfectly fine, thank you very much.

They are going about their day, thinking their happy thoughts, doing happy things, being quite all right.

They are the 1%.

Probably the 0.01%, really.

And good for them. Way to be the outliers.

This book isn't for them.

(Though they're welcome to read it. *Hello! We all float down here!*)

This book is for the rest of us — the 99.99%.

Because in the 21st century:

Being fucked up is normal.

Maybe that's not entirely comforting, and you really really wish you could be those nice 0.01% people, but at least you're not alone on the crazy train.

What wack shit are you doing?

Circle anything that's "Definitely me."

Put a star beside anything that doesn't apply... but does make you feel a little squicky when you read it.

Underline anything that makes you feel insulted, offended, or mad, like "Fuck you KSD, you don't know me!" Really press hard with the pen to let me know you mean business.

Often, I...

eat more than my body needs

eat less than my body needs

think about food a lot

think about eating or not-eating a lot

read about food / eating / diets

read about workout / exercise routines

feel hungry

want to eat... a lot

look at food- or body-related stuff on social media

feel like I'm not doing enough

have cravings

chew on stuff compulsively, like gum or ice chips

exercise until I feel exhausted or sore

feel tired or lethargic

have an upset stomach or poor digestion

34

feel smug and self-righteous about my diet — look at those ignorant dumbasses eating their shitty unhealthy food!

feel smug and self-righteous about my exercise — look at those lazy assholes lying on the couch!

say "No excuses" or "Harden up"

feel sad, anxious, and / or bad about my body

feel sad, anxious, and / or bad about my eating habits

deliberately harm myself or feel like pain is productive

feel irritable and angry

do things secretively, like sneak into the gym for more exercise, or hide food, or eat alone

feel anxious when I can't get the food I prefer

feel stressed out

feel alone

vomit, shit or otherwise try to purge or compensate for what I've eaten

make "rules" for myself

feel achey or sore

feel like I "lose control"

feel like I have to "get back in control"

touch / poke / pinch my body or look in the mirror to inspect flaws

vow to start again tomorrow, or on Monday

lie to other people about what I'm doing

want to change but can't seem to

wonder what the fuck is wrong with me

something else:

_____

(Almost) all of us are fucked up about food and eating.

Now, it's really important for me not to be an imperialist, egocentric dick here.

What I should say is:

Almost all of us living in Westernized, educated, industrialized, relatively rich, and democratic (aka WEIRD) parts of the globe are fucked up about food and eating.

So that's not everyone.

Other non-WEIRD folks tend to have different food and eating issues than WEIRD folks.

Like surviving famines, malnutrition, food scarcity, infected drinking water, armed rebels cutting off supplies, and stuff like that.

And of course, many people living in WEIRD countries have issues like not being able to afford food, or afford healthy food, or relying on food banks to get by.

It's all relative.

I don't mention this because I'm trying to make you feel bad or silly about your own situation, or guilty because someone else "has it worse".

I mention this to put things into perspective. And also, to give you a context for why you might feel the way you feel, and might do the things you do.

People living in WEIRD countries are experiencing things that humans *literally have never done or felt before.*

There's a lot of awesome stuff that happens in WEIRD places.

Like robot cars, central air conditioning that you can control with your phone, face transplants, doggie daycares, and whatnot.

But we've made some trade-offs for those advantages.

For instance, in historical terms, as a group:

- **We've never been so painfully aware of how we look, or how our bodies work.**

- **We've never had so much food, and so much tasty food.**

- **We've never had such high expectations for ourselves.**

- **We've never been so out of sync with our biology.**

- **We've never felt so alone.**

In particular, people in WEIRD countries, despite the "R", are more likely than non-WEIRD folks to say they feel:

- depressed;

- anxious;

- overwhelmed;

- stressed; and

- disconnected from other people.

It's weird — see what I did there? — because in WEIRD countries, we're surrounded by abundance.

We have all of the food.

We have all of the toys.

We have *all of the things*.

And yet.

Here we are.

In other words, you're normal.

If you struggle with food, and/or eating, and/or exercise, and/or body issues...

...join the club.

The Food and Eating and Exercise and Body Issues Club (FEEBIC) is not really a fun club — like, say, recreational beer league softball, or extreme quilting, or roller derby, or lazer disco bowling, or Roller Coaster Boggle (which isn't a thing, but should be).

But FEEBIC is not an elite club either. Most of us are in it.

There is no such thing as Everyone Else Who Is Better Than You.

Even if it seems like that.

There is no magical, special, gifted, perfect person who has it all figured out.

(Well except those 0.01% people. Fuck those assholes.)

In fact, the people who seem most magical, special, gifted, and "perfect" are often the most miserable.

Trust me on this one. I've seen behind the curtain.

What do you think everyone else is doing, thinking, or feeling right now?

Does it feel like "everyone else" has it together so much better than you?

If yes, how? If no, why not?

_____

_____

_____

_____

_____

_____

tRY DOODLING WHAt YOU
tHINK "NORMAL" LooKS LIKE.

tHEN RIP OUt tHIS PAGE.
CRUMPLE It UP.
AND SEt It ON FIRE.
FUCK NORMAL.

It's probably not about
the thing you think it's
about.

Aside from some basic advice, which I'll get to later on, issues with food and eating and not-eating and exercise and body image are almost never about just those things.

If they were, we could fix them much easier.

So:

There's no magic eating plan. (Although some are better than others. More on that later.)

There's no magic movement plan. (Although some are better than others. More on that later.)

There's no magic mindset. (Although... ah, never mind, you know what I'm going to say.)

There's no magic anything.

Thanks for nuthin, reality!

If you're fucked up, it's complicated. There's no quick fix and the fundamental issue often isn't where you expect it to be.

That doesn't mean you're doomed.

It just means that as human beings, we're all balls of string that need slow, caring, and patient un-tangling.

It also means that even if you work through your shit productively and maturely, you're still *you* at the end of it. And that's OK.

It's not your fault.

It's not your fault.

It's not your fault.

You need to know this.

Even if you don't feel it right now.

☆ IMAGINATION TIME! ☆

If it were true that your fuckedupitude was NOT your fault, how might that change things for you?

☐ **Ha! I already believe that.** Kumbaya KSD.

☐ **I refuse to believe that.** That removes free will. KSD, are you some kind of Commie?

☐ **I don't believe in imagination.** Fuck you KSD for asking me to use my right brain.

☐ **Why KSD! What an intriguing question!** Believing that my fuckedupitude is NOT my fault would mean...

_____

_____

_____

_____

OR, DOODLE WHAT MIGHT
CHANGE FOR YOU, IF YOUR
FUCKEDUPItUDE WAS NOt YOUR
FAULt.

THIS IS YOUR IMAGINAtION.
SO NO RULES.
BUt A SPARKLY UNICORN
WOULD GO GOOD HERE.

You are not broken.

You are not a failure.

You are not bad, stupid, weak, lazy, or immoral.

You do not have some terrible unique character flaw.

You are absolutely normal.

You are having a normal human reaction to some fucked up shit.

Actually, the fact that you're struggling with food and eating and exercise and body stuff shows that your magnificent resilient self is trying to help you.

It's trying to solve the problem.

It's trying to keep you safe from pain and trauma and fear and lots of bad stuff.

We'll talk more about this later.

Right now, though, you probably feel broken. So let's talk more about that.

Deep down, how do you think you *might* be completely, irrevocably broken?

☐   **Duh! You just said that I am not broken, KSD.** Are you fucking with me?

☐   **I have a few concerns, which I will list below...**

☐   **I'm going to need to sharpen a whole lot of pencils.** Here goes...

_____

_____

_____

_____

_____

_____

tRY DOODLING A PICtURE
OF WHAt YOUR BROKEN-NESS
WOULD LooK LIKE ON AN
X-RAY.

NOW DRAW IN SOME
SPLINtS, SCARS, AND StItCHES.
MAKE It looK REAL GROSS.

It's not your fault:
Trauma is a thing.

You know what the biggest factors in people's fuckedupitude are?

Trauma and stress.

For instance, research shows that people who've been abused emotionally, physically, and/or sexually are more likely to have issues with food, eating/not-eating, exercise, and/or body image.

But it doesn't have to be "big-T" Trauma like emotional abuse, or rape, or violence, to affect you.

It can be "little-t" trauma. The daily bullshit and emotional paper cuts of everyday life.

Relationships. Finances.

Moving. Other transitions. Feeling adrift and lost.

Not having a clear sense of self.

Feeling alone.

Shame. Grief. Loss.

Sexism. Racism. Homophobia. Ageism.

All the other "isms" and insults that eventually just sort of form a toxic sludge that we swim in and get up our noses.

We're soaking in it.

Trauma lives in our bodies.

Trauma and distress make their presence known even if we aren't consciously aware of them.

Our bodies tell the truth.

Our bodies record our history.

As psychotherapist Bessel van der Kolk aptly puts it, the body keeps the score.

Bodies can't speak in words.

Bodies speak in pain. Or trying to kill the pain.

Bodies speak in movements and body language. Like tightness or bracing or rigidity or freezing or shrinking down into a little ball of shame.

Bodies speak in energy — whether that's a frantic perma-busyness and anxious fidgeting, or lethargy and exhaustion and hopelessness.

Bodies speak in food and eating / not-eating and appetite and cravings and never feeling full and wanting to chew everything and either avoiding or chasing the hollow feeling of emptiness.

Bodies speak in the desire to purge, to retch, to shit, to claw skin off, to heave and spew the toxic garbage of the world and all the feelings that burn like battery acid inside.

What's the earliest memory you have of being fucked up in the way you are now?

For instance, if you over-eat, when was the first time you remember doing that? Or, if you under-eat, when was the first time you remember doing that? Or...?

_____

_____

_____

_____

_____

_____

OR, DOODLE A PICTURE OF YOUR EARLIEST MEMORY OF BEING FUCKED UP IN THE WAY YOU ARE NOW.

LIKE: "HERE'S ME HIDING FOOD WHEN I WAS 6." OR: "HERE'S ME GOING ON A DIET WITH MY MOM WHEN I WAS 12."

FEEL FREE TO CRY A LITTLE BIT RIGHT NOW. THIS SHIT IS FUCKING SAD. SEE IF YOU CAN MAKE SOME TEAR STAINS HERE.

Start with one breath.

Fuckedupitude happens when we don't have other, better tools to deal with things.

It's like trying to build a house when you only have a sledgehammer. A sledgehammer works great for a few tasks, and feels good to swing, but mostly smashes shit.

So let's add a tool here. It's a breath.

Remember: Stuff lives in your body.

Let's start teaching your body that there are other options. Here's how.

Breathe in. Just a regular breath, no fancy stuff.

Breathe out. Slow. Reallll slow. Like you are blowing up a big balloon.

Empty your lungs as much as you can. Try to squeak out a little more air. Make a lung sandwich. Squish your lungs between your ribs and your guts and your spine.

Pause. Just for a few seconds.

Relax and let yourself breathe in naturally. Don't huff. Don't force it. Just let your lungs do their thing. They know their job.

That's it.

Try that a few more times. And whenever you feel kinda freaked out by this book.

Talk to your monster.

You can't leave a place you've never been.

You've probably avoided *really* looking at your fuckedupitude, even though it might be dominating your life.

(And that makes sense. Who the fuck wants to look at this shit?)

If you want to move away from your fuckedupitude, you have to actually stop there and look around for a while.

Whatever your inner monster is, it won't go away if you ignore it.

You have to sit down on the couch with your monster and have a little chat. Get to know it. Hang out with it.

I know, I know.

Gross.

Euw.

Ugh.

Let's get through this together.

Try a couple of those lung-sandwich breathing things from the previous page first.

If you could talk to the monster inside of you, what would it say?

_____

_____

_____

_____

_____

_____

_____

OR, DOODLE THE MONSTER
THAT LIVES INSIDE OF YOU.

THEN MAKE THE SOUND IT WOULD MAKE.

Pause now.

Talking to your monster is some heavy shit.

Don't try to do it all at once.

Take a break.

Take a lung-sandwich breath.

Do that thing little kids do with their tongue where they go *bla-dle-la-dle-la-dle*.

Take another lung-sandwich breath.

Go get a foot rub, or a glass of water, or something.

INtERM

ISSION!!!

Where does the problem NOT happen?

As crazy as it sounds:

Your life isn't 100% fucked.

Simple mathematics tells us that we can't be wack all the time.

For instance, let's say you're someone who feels like they constantly think about food.

Like, all day long, 24/7.

Wake up for a pee in the middle of the night, and as you shamble the bathroom you think about food, or eating, or body stuff.

This was me once.

But if we *actually catalogued each and every one of your thoughts and feelings,* we would find that not all of them are about food.

Try it yourself. For 10 minutes, write down every thought you have.

You might find that lots of them are about whether you should let the dog out, or your taxes, or whether you should turn up the thermostat, or whatever.

Another example:

If you binge eat for a few hours every day, you still have hours in the day when you are *not* bingeing.

Let's imagine your day looks like this:

    7 AM - Wake up
    9 AM - 5 PM - Work
    6 PM - 11 PM - Binge eat
    11 PM - 7 AM - Sleep

Even if you binge for 5 hours a day, every day, you are still *not* bingeing for 19 hours a day.

In other words, you are NOT bingeing about 75% of the time.

And even if you say "Well, 11 PM to 7 AM, I'm asleep, and I feel pretty crappy when I wake up, and my stomach doesn't stop being upset until around noon…"

Even if we could say that *up to 18 hours a day* is either binge eating or binge recovering…

…that's still not 100% of the time.

Flip your perspective and look for where the problem is NOT happening.

This is where you will find your clues about how to change.

Where and when does the problem NOT happen?

Where and when are things better for you, even just a little bit?

_____

_____

_____

_____

_____

_____

_____

Meet your resilient self.

Right now, you may feel weak and empty and depleted and afraid.

So you do not believe in such things as resilient selves or that you have one.

But you do.

You have a strong, resilient, persistent, survivor-self within you.

Take a breath. Feel the air. Life is pumping in and out of your lungs. Touch your neck or your wrists. Feel your pulse thumping through your veins.

If you cut yourself, your body will try to heal you *even if you don't want it to*.

Life proceeds.

Your body converts a pile of random chemicals into YOU. Over and over and over.

Holy fuck. Isn't that amazing.

Your resilient self is the part of you that whispers *I'm not dead yet, assholes*.

As long as you can exchange oxygen for carbon dioxide, and move those red blood cells from downstairs to upstairs, some part of you will always seek survival and healing and wholeness.

This may feel confusing.

If we all have a resilient self — a self that seeks wholeness, and healing, and growth, and life — why are we all fucked up?

Why do we do things that don't seem to make sense?

Like why do we start our day vowing to be better, and end our day face-down in ice cream?

Like why do we vow that we will *totally* change on Monday, and by Saturday (or maybe Tuesday) we are (hopefully figuratively) shitting the bed?

Like why do we find ourselves doing stuff we swore we would never do again? Maybe 30 seconds afterwards?

You know what I mean.

It's a great big what the fuck.

It's like we're on autopilot sometimes, and that autopilot seems to be set to *Crash and Burn*.

It *is* confusing.

Blame your brain. And the world around you.

Remember, it's not your fault.

There's often something good about being "bad".

Often, our fuckeduptitude started out kinda fun.

Or it helped us get through a tough time. It was a tool to fix something.

Or it was originally a good idea. Like trying to eat healthier, or get into shape.

Somehow our brains got the idea:

Certain choices are rewarding.

Our brains get a little shot of *Woohoo!* every time we make those choices. Our brains, being smart, learn fast: *Do that again. Seek it out.*

Soon, our brains are looking for those choices everywhere.

After a while, stuff that *was* fun, or *was* working, *was* originally a good idea, sometimes stops being fun or workable or a good idea. But sometimes... it still feels kinda valuable, too.

Important: This isn't about blame.

I'm not saying you *enjoy* being fucked up.

In fact, that's the problem. If you completely enjoyed being fucked up, you wouldn't be reading this book. You'd be off partying with celebrities, getting ready to die in a drunken naked skydiving accident.

In fact, some stuff feels terrific.

I'll be honest with you.

I enjoyed many things about my fuckedupitude.

Tearing through a buffet.

The delicious, decadent pleasure of eating whatever I wanted, as much as I wanted. 'Cause I'm a grownup! Yeah! I'll eat that entire jar of peanut butter because FUCK YOU!

Self-righteousness. Feeling smug because I thought I had all The Diet & Workout Secrets.

Liking the feeling of being hungry because I thought it meant I was *getting ripped*. That I was better and more disciplined than everyone else.

Sweet, sweet stress relief. Kicking back. Relaxing with a nice big plate of *aaaaaahhhhh*.

Watching my abs emerge, stripped by starvation. Modestly receiving compliments on how great my arms looked.

Walking around the city late at night, randomly buying stoner food from bodegas. I felt like this one made me a real *bon vivant*.

Not giving a fuck after a long week of giving too many fucks.

Food comas.

Secretly, what feels good or useful or helpful about what you're currently doing?

☐ It helps me cope with:

_____.

☐ It helps me forget about:

_____.

☐ It feels good because:

_____.

☐ It gives me:

_____.

☐ I enjoy that:

_____.

☐ Some other reason:

_____

_____

_____

DOODLE WHAT THE MOST
AWESOME!! PART OF YOUR
FUCKEDUPITUDE IS.

RUB THIS SHEET ON YOUR BRAIN.
OOOHHH YEAH.

There are damn good reasons NOT to change.

Change sucks.

It's hard.

It's uncomfortable.

It means leaving behind a system that we've carefully built and tended.

It means facing new things. Scary things.

It means taking risks.

It means losing our security blanket.

It means giving up the only barrier that we feel is standing between us and *total chaos*.

It means grief.

You know what we call sudden, fast, forced change that overwhelms our ability to cope with it?

Trauma.

That's how shitty change is.

Fuck change.

What would suck about changing?

☐ I would have to give up:

_____.

☐ I would lose:

_____.

☐ I would have to face:

_____.

☐ I would have to learn to:

_____.

☐ I would grieve:

_____.

☐ Some other bullshit:

_____

_____

_____

DOODLE tHE **COMPLEtE FUCKING DISAStER** tHAt WOULD OCCUR IF YOU DID, IN FACt, CHANGE.

HERE ARE FLAMES. YOUR LIFE IS ON FIRE BECAUSE YOU CHANGED!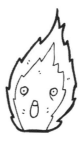

It's not your fault:
Your brain hides things
from you.

Your brain is sneaky. It *feels* like you're aware of everything it's thinking and doing.

But you're not.

Your brain hides a lot of things from you.

It's not trying to be a douche. It's just that if you had to pay attention to every single brain function from tying your shoes to remembering to breathe, you wouldn't be able to do anything.

So most of your thinking and feeling is below the radar.

Most of your behaviour is automatic.

Habitual. You do it without thinking.

Which is the point.

Actively *thinking* takes effort.

But automatic thoughts, feelings, and behaviours don't.

That's how your brain likes it. Easy peasy.

For most of what you think, feel, and do, your brain can just press the button marked "Habit", then kick back in a lawn chair and relax as you run through your pre-programmed sequence.

That's a great strategy... until it's not.

Ever driven somewhere familiar, not really paying attention, and then you arrived, and you realized you'd driven the entire way with almost no memory of what just happened?

How the hell did you not crash the car?

Ever had an eating episode where you just kind of "zoned out", and basically woke up in a pile of crumbs and empty containers?

How the hell did you get your hand to your mouth, chew, and swallow without choking?

That's the power of your automatic brain.

Once it learns where and how to get rewards, your automatic brain will purposely hijack:

- **your attention** (so your attention gets directed towards all things food / eating / not-eating / exercise / compensating)

- **your focus** (so that the entire universe shrinks to your pursuit of your fucked up shit)

- **your memory** (so you forget about what you're doing, or how painful it is, or how often you do it)

- **your reasoning and decison making** (so that it seems *completely logical* to use a party-sized pizza as a burrito wrap and throw some chocolate chips on top)

Once you're in the habit of getting rewards, your brain starts to look for reward cues everywhere: in the grocery store, at the office, under the couch.

Where's the tasty food that'll soothe me?

Where's the new diet that'll fix me?

Where's the kickass booty-boosting exercise plan?

Where's the social media feed full of food and lifestyle porn and happy beautiful fit people?

It's all cues, all the time.

On top of that, your brain starts actively ignoring other stuff.

Like non-food, non-exercise cues. Like positive information such as *You look perfectly fine.* Like other people desperately trying to connect with you, because they feel alone too.

When you get cued or triggered under the right circumstances, you become a finely tuned fuckedupitude execution machine.

But *you don't know it.*

Your automatic brain engages the automatic pilot, making you do automatic things.

All you know is that it kinda feels like being dragged behind a psychotic horse as it runs wildly towards an ice cream sundae.

Your fuckedupitude is trying to *help* you. (Poorly.)

It may seem like your brain and body and behaviours are out to get you.

Like they exist purely to ruin your life.

Look at this motherfucker wanting more food! You stupid asshole!

Look at me doing the same goddamned stupid thing again! What the fuck?!

And so on.

In fact, your brain and body and behaviours are trying to *help* you.

To protect you. To keep you safe. To soothe your stress. To numb and mask your pain.

To distract you from terror, and shame, and loneliness, and sadness, and anger. To keep you feeling good, or at least sane.

Of course, your brain and body and behaviours are probably doing more harm than good now.

They're like a well-meaning but misguided and socially awkward friend.

Your friend loves you.

Your friend tries to help... but they muddle things up.

Ironically, you stop enjoying the reward.

The definition of an addiction is continuing to seek out a reward compulsively, *even though that reward might not even be all that fun any more.*

All behaviour is an attempt to solve a problem.

Our habits work for us, until they don't.

At one time, whatever you did worked for you, more or less. It solved a problem, or tried to.

Now, maybe your behaviours don't work so well for you. They might cost you a lot these days.

(Even if they might sometimes still be valuable or fun or a good emotional anesthetic.)

We often stop liking what we're doing.

But we don't stop seeking it out.

This is because "liking" and "wanting" are two different systems in our brains.

We can *want* something — maybe even feel obsessed by it — even if we don't really *like* it.

Ha ha! Oh brain! You and your shenanigans!

How is your fuckedupitude NOT working for you?

What are your thoughts, feelings, and behaviours costing you? What are their consequences? How do they harm you or work against what you want?

_____

_____

_____

_____

_____

_____

_____

DOODLE WHAT COULD HAPPEN
IF YOU KEEP GOING LIKE
YOU'RE GOING FOR ANOTHER
10 OR 20 YEARS.

Get off autopilot.

This is easier said than done.

But now you know:

Your brain has an autopilot.

That autopilot is *designed* to keep you unaware of its operation.

Now you can start changing how often and how much you use that autopilot.

But first, we are just going to do two things:

1. Notice what is happening.

2. Name it.

(If we can.)

This might be hard to notice, at first.

Of course, you might not know what situations trigger you, or make you feel crappy. It's the ol' brain *Don't look behind the curtain routine*.

Don't worry if it feels tricky at first.

You *can* start paying attention.

You *can* start learning.

You *can* start mapping out the terrain of your experiences.

Here's how.

Every time you have an upsetting or stressful thought or feeling...

Every time you make a choice that doesn't feel like your best, most highly evolved, most self-compassionate, wisest, or most resilient self is driving...

Every time you do something you regret...

Every time you feel like shit is falling apart...

...jot down a few notes.

That's all.

Over time, you'll start to see patterns. Something is connected to something else.

Look for familiar scripts and stories.

Here's a funny paradox about trying to name what you are noticing.

(Funny strange, not funny ha-ha.)

If words about feelings or thoughts or experiences or situations seem clear and clean and sure and swift... *those words might be wrong.*

Here's an example. Your coworker gives you the side-eye. You immediately jump to an explanation that feels rock-solid: *Coworker is an insensitive jerk!*

That story seems crystal clear. And so very correct.

But it's not. Your coworker was actually looking out the window behind you.

Your fast and powerful assumption was wrong.

Even if it *felt right,* because it came so quickly and clearly.

The reason it felt so fast and true was that *you were just replaying a familiar script* instead of *actually describing what was really happening* in that moment.

Maybe years ago you learned: *People are jerks.* Now you look at everything through jerk-coloured glasses.

Our lives are full of familiar scripts and stories.

Like beloved fairy tales or movies you watch a million times, we know those scripts and stories well — every line, every plot twist, every conflict, every character.

We use scripts and stories to try to explain the world.

They're sort of like rules about How Things Work.

Remember our brain shorthand?

Unless we've trained our minds to *enjoy* (or at least tolerate) ambiguity and complexity, they don't like when things seem confusing, or unclear, or don't seem to make sense.

Our minds are like those professional organizers that charge $150 an hour to colour-code and alphabetize and sort all your crap into tidy boxes.

If something is out of place, our minds try to jam it into a mental box.

No loose ends! No tangles!

We like things to follow the scripts. And we follow the scripts too.

Here are some sample scripts.

See if any of these sound like the movies in your head. **Circle** the ones that are familiar. (It's OK if none of them fit you.)

I can't do anything right.

I should...

Everyone is out to get me.

You can't trust people.

I try hard, but I always fuck things up.

Things were fine, until...

Fuck it. I'm tired of all this hard work.

It's one damn thing after another.

I feel like I'm on a treadmill, and I can't get off.

People always disappoint me.

It's better not to get too close to people.

If I keep working hard, I'll get somewhere.

I'm so tired.

Stuff just seems to happen to me.

I'm so overwhelmed.

I'm just fucked up, I guess.

I'm doomed. Nothing can help me.

I'm such a crybaby sometimes.

I work so hard and nobody appreciates that.

It never feels like "enough".

Here are some sample characters you could play in the movie of your life.

Circle the ones that sound familiar.

X out the ones that piss you off in your own life.

The Crybaby

The Get Shit Done Person

The Sufferer

The Awkward Dork

The Loner

The Misunderstood

The Fraud

The Brilliant Success

The Caretaker

The High Roller

The Achiever

The Fuckup

The Good Friend With A Great Personality

The Smartypants

The Hot Chick / Dude

The Freedom Fighter

The Giver

The Janitor (Who Mops Up Someone Else's Mess All The Goddamned Time)

The Popular Girl / Guy

The Know-It-All

The Lost & Confused

The Hero / Heroine

The Tells-It-Like-It-Is Straight Shooter

Who else could you play?

Write down other characters that you might play in the movie of your life.

OR, DOODLE A PICTURE OF YOUR CHARACTER.

Play in the mud.

As we've seen, if explanations about the world come too easily, they may be wrong. We may just be reviewing a familiar script, in which we play familiar characters, instead of actually explaining what's happening in the moment.

Here's the corollary of that:

If words about feelings or thoughts or experiences or situations are mucky and muddy and slow and searching... those words might be *right*.

Have you ever struggled to explain a vague or unclear sensation, like a weird feeling you got about someone?

"I mean, he seems OK... but... I dunno... there's just something about him... I can't quite put my finger on it... He's polite and everything... but..."

You can't seem to find the words to capture your sense of things.

But you know there is a *feeling*. There is a deep, intuitive sensation that wants to be heard and acknowledged.

Words here feel inadequate. Garbled. Hard to find. You can't quite describe what is happening, but you know that *something is*.

That's what we're looking for. Playing in the mud.

Use your imagination.

Remember English class, where you learned about metaphors and similes? Well now we're actually going to use that stuff you thought you would never use.

Also remember that our bodies don't speak in words? Words are hard to find when we're describing deep, powerful, gut-level rumblings that we need to pay attention to.

So we use sensations and images instead.

Now you get to use your imagination!

Here's how.

Sit down quietly.

Mentally "scan" your body from head to toe.

Observe any sensations that you discover, but don't judge them. You are being curious here, not critical.

Sit with those sensations for a few seconds.

See if you can make an image out of them. Start with, "It's like..." and then wait. (I've given you some ideas on the next page.)

Wait some more. This is slow.

Try an image again. Wait.

If you settle on an image that seems to fit, write it down or draw it to record it.

"When I scan my body, it's like..."

Try these images on and see if they fit.

Or come up with your own.

...a rhino is sitting on my chest.

...my pants are full of spiders.

...I just want to punch something.

...my head feels like a soggy cotton ball.

...my heart is smashing its way out of my chest with its fists.

...my stomach is tied up in knots.

...my eyes have been sandpapered.

...all the air is gone.

...if I start crying, it'll be a flood.

...my chest is full of happy bubbles.

...my skin is much too tight. I am a human sausage.

...a thousand bees are stinging my spine.

...my sinuses are full of lead.

...I weigh ten thousand pounds.

...I am floating.

...I want to run for the exit.

...I could kick the world in the ass with my ENERGY LEGS!!!

...I am dissolving from the inside out.

NOW YOU TRY IT.

"WHEN I SCAN MY BODY, IT'S LIKE..."
DRAW OR WRITE DOWN WHAT COMES
NEXT.

Slow ya roll.

Slowness is your friend.

The more you slow down and pay attention:

- the more you'll be able to notice what's really going on.

- the more you'll be able to match what you do to what you really, truly, deeply want.

- the more you'll feel in charge of your choices.

- the more you'll feel like you can be wise, calm, thoughtful, and purposeful.

Now, I don't mean ruminate and over-think and grind your mental gears.

I mean *pause*.

Look around. Take a breath.

You didn't get here overnight and you won't fix things overnight.

Let yourself move slowly.

Slowing down is hard nowadays.

So if you have the guts to slow the fuck down while everyone else is flailing and panicked, you're a rebel! You're badass! You're a trailblazer!

Cool!

Start noticing what's around you.

We evolved to take cues from our environment.

Even bacteria follow environmental cues: hot, cold, acid, alkaline, delicious poop or raw meat to munch on, and so on.

Unless you're in a coma, you are *always* observing and responding to things and people around you.

But most of the time, *you don't realize it.*

So, for instance, if you're getting a brain reward from over-eating, you're not just getting the hit from simply chewing and swallowing.

You're also getting a reward from things like:

- **where you are** (maybe at home, chilling out?)

- **the package** (shiny! colourful!)

- **smells** (Cinnabon amirite?!)

- **who you're with** (your BBBF — best binge buddy forever?)

- **the situation** (party night out with the boys or girls? alone after a tough day at work?)

- **the hunt** (finding that treat, thinking about finding that treat, imagining eating that treat...)

Think about whatever you are doing in your own life that is related to food, eating / not-eating, exercise and body image.

Now think about the situations that you might be in when things feel worse, more upsetting, and / or more out of control.

☐   I over-eat / binge when:

_____.

☐   I under-eat / restrict food when:

_____.

☐   I try to control my food / eating when:

_____.

☐   I feel anxious about things when:

_____.

☐   I feel cravings when:

_____.

☐   I do some other shit when:

_____

DOODLE tHE SItUAtIONS tHAt MAKE YOU FEEL **WORSt** OR MOSt CRAZY.

Now flip that.

What's around us can encourage us to feel worse.

What's around us can also help us feel, and be, and do, better.

Go back to the previous exercise and flip it.

Think about the situations, people, and environments that:

- care about you

- encourage you

- calm you

- focus you

- make you feel truly good

- inspire you

- excite you

- fulfill you

- support you

- help you be your best self

If you don't have many of those in real life, imagine what they *could* be.

Think about whatever you are doing in your own life that is related to food, eating / not-eating, exercise and body image.

Now think about the situations that you might be in when things feel better, calmer, happier, wiser, supportive, and / or more purposeful.

☐ I feel purposeful when:

_____.

☐ I feel good about my choices when:

_____.

☐ I feel content when:

_____.

☐ I feel relaxed and calm when:

_____.

☐ I feel supported when:

_____.

☐ I feel inspired when:

_____

DOODLE tHE SItuAtIONS tHAt MAKE YOU FEEL **BESt** OR MOSt AWESOME.

REMEMBER, IF YOU DON't HAVE tHESE IN REAL LIFE, YOU CAN StARt BY JUSt IMAGINING tHEM...

DOUBLE INTERM

FUCKIN' ISSION!!!

YOU EARNED It.

Only action creates change.

OK, we've been doing lots of heavy thinking and feeling and remembering and noticing.

That's great. That's important.

It's good to look before you leap. In fact, I highly recommend that as a life strategy.

At the same time:

If you want things to be different, you eventually have to *do something*.

You have to take action.

Now, that action doesn't have to be big.

In fact, it probably shouldn't be.

But it has to be *something*.

Action creates power.

Along with wrecking our health, sanity, and relationships, issues with food and eating and not-eating and exercise and body image make us feel powerless.

We feel immobilized and helpless. We feel hopeless and lost.

Eventually, this becomes normal.

We assume we *really are* helpless and hopeless and stupid and shitty and a lost cause.

But we aren't.

We are more powerful than we can imagine... *if we take action.*

Your strongest weapon against fuckedupitude is *doing something*.

Action *creates* power.

Action *creates* growth.

Action *creates* clarity.

Action *creates* confidence.

Action *creates* motivation. (Not the other way round.)

We can behave our way into being something else.

Something fresh, and new, and amazing, and free.

Little movements make big movements.

Ever watch pro wrestling?

It's full of big, acrobatic, theatrical movements.

Giant flips, lifting other people overhead then flinging them to the mat, leaping out of the ring, wildly swinging a folding chair *Oh my God I can't believe the ref is allowing that...*

Well, real wrestling, and real life, is usually not like that.

More often, we find ourselves mashed into a very undignified position, unable to escape.

At that point, it's easy to panic or feel hopeless. Especially when our big moves don't work, or we can't do them.

My wrestling teacher once told me: "Little movements make big movements."

What that means is that if you're stuck in a bad spot, try wriggling out, millimetre by millimetre, being patient and persistent.

Wriggle one: One millimetre.

Wriggle two: Two millimetres.

And so on. Tiny changes start adding up.

Then suddenly, you're free!

Now it's time to grab that folding chair to get revenge.

What's your little movement?

Let's say you're ready to make a move.

(You don't actually have to be. But let's say, hypothetically, that you are.)

You've decided that you want to take some kind of action towards change.

You realize that you're tired of thinking, and worrying, and wondering, and doing a whole bunch of other stuff that doesn't get you anywhere.

Just making this decision is incredibly courageous.

So pause (see! we slow down!) and recognize the bravery of even considering doing something different.

Now, ask yourself:

What's the next move I can make?

What's the *tiniest, laziest, easiest, low-hanging-fruitiest* thing I could do to move in a new and positive direction?

What can I do to start wriggling out of this chokehold, millimetre by millimetre?

It's OK if you aren't sure yet. Just start thinking about it.

Seriously, like really little movements.

People often get poopyface or disappointed when I don't have the Big Hairy Answer for them (what I call the Magic Bean — the thing that will magically solve all your problems immediately).

The truth is, we need to keep our change-actions very, very, *very* small.

Big change, done too quickly, is trauma.

We've all had enough of that shit.

Big changes tend not to stick.

We've all had enough of that shit too.

Think micro-changes.

No, think nano-changes. Or even smaller.

(Fun fact! The prefix for a "one-septillionth" is "yocto". So we're talking about yocto-changes. Or, if you're feeling ambitious today, try a zepto-change or atto-change, which are one-sextillionth or one-quintillionth, respectively.)

When deciding on change, here's the sound I listen for: *Pff*.

In Canada, we call this a "flat tire". It's the sound of a tire quickly deflating, as in, "I asked Maureen to the prom, and she totally flat-tired me." It's a sound of amused disbelief, like *Are you shitting me?*

When considering how big your change-action should be, you're looking for the flat-tire level of indulgent but dismissive judgement, like this:

Pff, are you serious, that is so easy.

Pff, I can totally do that blindfolded.

Pff, you must be joking, I did that ten times today already.

Whatever change-action you are proposing, it must feel hilariously, stupidly, frustratingly, ridiculously easy and do-able under any conditions.

This, of course, is the opposite of what we normally do.

Which is taking on giant, unrealistic, soul-crushing projects that inevitably crash and burn, leaving us feeling like hot wet baby-diaper garbage.

This doesn't mean big changes are *always* bad.

Big changes happen whether we want them to or not.

Sometimes, big changes are terrific.

Like finally leaving a shitty job, or a shitty partner, or a shitty living situation.

Like piling into your car with a dog to go to some weird psychedelic art festival *even though you don't own a dog.*

Like saying an unexpected "Yes" or "No" that you would normally *never* say. ("Yes! Give me that face tattoo! What the hell!")

But again, much of the time, big changes are difficult, painful, traumatic, and hard to sustain.

The secret to the flat-tire level of E-Zy change is:

You are guaranteed to succeed.

The more you succeed, the better you feel.

The better you feel, the more you want to do.

The more you want to do, the more you *can* do.

Here are some of the adjectives that could apply to the actions you try.

simple

fun

manageable

easy

lazy

basic

effortless

obvious

natural

familiar

straightforward

uncomplicated

reasonable

child's play

no sweat

light

little

like falling off a log (this may be a Canadianism)

a cinch

a snap

a doddle (for my UK friends)

painless

quick

something I do anyway

nothing to it

elementary

attainable

manageable

do-able

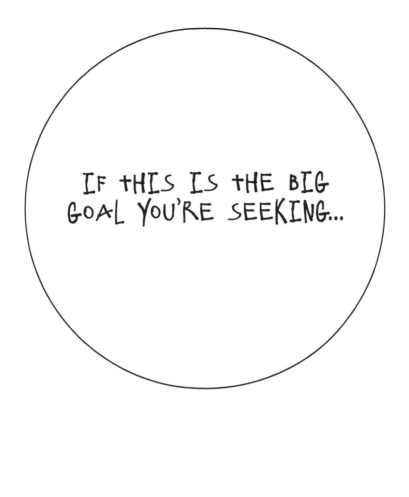

IF tHIS IS tHE BIG GOAL YOU'RE SEEKING...

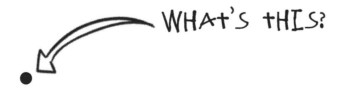

WHAt'S tHIS?

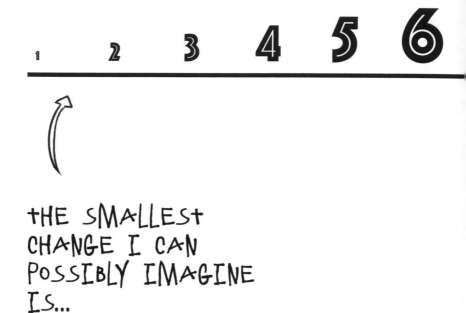

THE SMALLEST
CHANGE I CAN
POSSIBLY IMAGINE
IS...

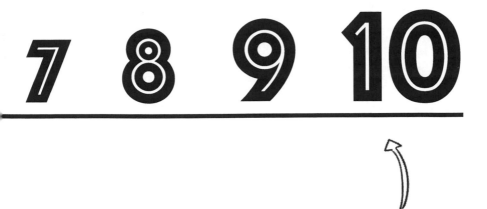

THE BIGGEST CHANGE
I CAN POSSIBLY
IMAGINE IS...

Just do *more* good things.

Look for what's already working... and just do more of it.

I know, I know. You probably want to slap me right now.

But stop and think. (There's that slowing-down thing again.)

Normally, don't we always focus on fixing mistakes? And improving "weaknesses"? And hiding or avoiding "failures"?

When was the last time you noticed:

- **what was *already* working?**

- **what was *already* good?**

- **what was *not* a fuckup?**

We tend to focus on the one plane crash rather than the eleven million that *don't* crash.

News would be pretty boring if it reported reality accurately.

"Most folks got home from work safely today."

"Millions of people were not poisoned by their drinking water / salad greens / nemesis."

"Even more millions of people don't even *have* a nemesis."

"Just do more good things" isn't some Pollyanna "think positive" bullshit.

"Do more of what is already working" is a damn good action plan.

Conversely, "Don't do X" is a terrible action plan.

You can't learn to drive by having someone tell you about how driving *isn't* fishing, and it *isn't* cooking, and you *don't* put your hands on the roof, and you *don't* sit in the trunk.

Well, what the fuck *do* you do, then?

You still don't know.

But let's say you're learning to drive, and you're with someone who simply focuses on getting you to do more of what is already working.

> "You're checking your mirrors well. Keep doing that, and add a little extra check before you change lanes."

> "I like how you're braking smoothly instead of slamming it down. See if you can make it even a little smoother."

> "Now you're starting to anticipate obstacles and slowdowns. Can you look even a little further ahead, to anticipate even more?"

Now learning to drive — which could have been terribly stressful and demoralizing — is almost getting fun.

More importantly, you have a clear sense of *what to do*.

When you:

- **look for what is already working** (or at least, a little bit better or further along the path you want to go); and

- **think about how to do or get more of that good stuff...**

...you have a blueprint for action.

Look for patterns.

Go back to the exercises where you captured the situations, people, and environments that make you feel things like:

- better

- calmer

- happier

- wiser

- supported

- purposeful

- inspired

- saner

- understood

- respected

- cared for

- awesome (or "brilliant" for my UK pals)

See if you can figure out what it is about those situations, people, and/or environments that makes them that way.

What, specifically, goes well?

Why, specifically, do those things make you feel better?

Who makes you feel best, and why?

List 3 people, real or imagined, who float your boat.

_____ makes me feel good (or inspired, or cared for, or whatever) because:

_____.

_____ makes me feel good (or inspired, or cared for, or whatever) because:

_____.

_____ makes me feel good (or inspired, or cared for, or whatever) because:

_____.

What makes you feel best, and why?

List 3 situations, real or imagined, that put you at your best (or at least a little better).

_____ makes me feel good (or proud, or competent, or whatever) because:

_____.

_____ makes me feel good (or proud, or competent, or whatever) because:

_____.

_____ makes me feel good (or proud, or competent, or whatever) because:

_____.

⚔ RESILIENT SELF AT WORK ⚔

You've probably tried many things in the past to change, grow, get better, or relieve suffering.

This is your resilient self at work.

List all the things you've tried.

(Think hard. There are probably more than you expect.)

☺ **Draw a happy face** beside the ones that worked best, were most successful, and / or truly felt like the best fit for you... even if they didn't last.

✓ **Draw a checkmark** beside the ones that didn't work all that well, but which taught you something. Learning is good!

To do things better, and/or to grow, and/or to change, I have tried...

_____

_____

_____

_____

_____

_____

_____

_____

_____

Now you have clues.

Once you've done the exercises on the previous pages (and feel free to do even more exploration of what is already working), you've got some clues.

What situations, people, and environments make things better, even *just a little bit*?

What do those things have in common?

How can you get or do more of that?

How have you *already* tried to change, grow, and improve?

What has *already* worked?

What have you *already* learned about yourself and what you need?

Put the thinking cap on and start noodling.

Are you ready?

Are you willing and able to do that teeny tiny positive action right now?

(Feel free to take time if you're not. I'll still be here.)

In the Ultimate Fighting Championship, I love how the referee asks both opponents:

Are you ready?

Are you ready?

And then the ref will yell:

LET'S GET IT ONNNNNN!!!

So, whenever your answer to "Are you ready?" is yes... turn the page.

Yelling *LET'S GET IT ONNNNNN!!!* is optional, but highly recommended.

Even better, see if you can find a giant dude with a booming baritone to do it for you.

(Unless you are *already* a giant dude with a booming baritone. Then you are your own ref.)

Do something.

Fucking DO IT!

Do the thing that you want to do!

The thing that is a teeny, tiny vote for change!

The thing that is easy and fun and feels great and drops a coin into your soul bank account!

DO IT!

Then you're done.

You can't un-do the thing you just did.

You now have inarguable evidence that *you can act in the service of your own change*.

Ha ha! Who's fucked up and hopeless now?!

Not you, that's for fucking sure.

Do another thing later.

Tomorrow, or later today. Or whenever.

Take one more thing like the thing you just did and do that second thing.

Keep acting in very, very, very small ways.

Every action is a drop of water.

If you think one drop of water is no big deal, consider this:

Would you like a drop of water on your pants right around crotch level?

How about a drop of coffee?

Would you like a drop of *a stranger's water on your face, knowing it came from some part of their body*?

Yeah. A drop doesn't seem so insignificant now, does it?

Imagine how fucking gross it would be to get *fourteen* drops of a stranger's uninvited body-water on your face.

Well, fourteen drops is two weeks of one action done every day.

Drops add up.

Or, more accurately...

**Actions don't just add.
They multiply.**

Change isn't like basic arithmetic, where you just add one action to one action to one action and so on.

I mean, not to knock arithmetic. (Shout out to my ancient Indian, Arab, Mayan, Egyptian, and Babylonian peeps! Good work on the zero.)

Change is actually more like something that scales exponentially.

Each change action makes the next change action *more likely* to happen.

So it's usually not like this:

$$1 + 1 + 1 + 1 + 1 + 1$$

It's usually more like this:

$$1 + 1 + 2 + 1 + 3 + 2 + 3 + 5 + 14 \text{ woohoo!}$$

Maybe you throw a 0.5 in there or whatever.

But the concept is the same.

I've got nice pictures of cats on the next page if you hate math.

To think about this another way:

Let's say you don't like cats.

You don't have a cat. You don't want a cat.

You're crabby and you hate everything.

But then... one day, you hear a noise outside your door.

You look. It's the most tiny, adorable, lovable kitten ever.

You bring the kitten inside.

You feed it. It's hungry. It makes adorable little licking and mewling sounds as it gobbles.

Your cat-hating heart of steel melts a little bit.

You mean to bring the kitten to the Humane Society, but... it's so damn cute.

Maybe you'll keep that cat another day.

Somewhere inside you, something's changed because you took this action.

You're not a cat lover... yet. But you at least don't hate this *particular* kitten.

So now, your household looks like this:

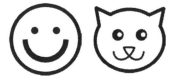

The kitten grows. Every day you do a few small actions, like feeding it, or playing with it.

You get to know it. You get to like it.

More importantly, *you build a habit of taking care of it*.

Every action you take to care for that kitten reinforces the fact that that kitten is valuable and deserves love.

One day, another stray cat scratches at your door.

This one's not as cute. It's more catty and less kitten-y.

Honestly, it looks a little scruffy and mangy.

But hey, now you have one cat... and you're taking care of it... so another cat is probably fine...

Now your house is like this:

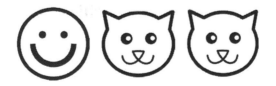

Every action you took made the next one possible... *and more likely.*

Eventually your house is like this:

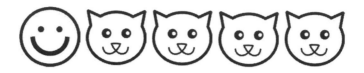

Because you built a habit of taking care of that first adorable kitten, you now have a menagerie of animals that you love and care for.

(And you're technically now a crazy cat lady / guy. But let's skip that part of the analogy.)

So what's the lesson here?

Take care of the thing you *hate the least*, at first.

Imagine some part of yourself, or your life, or the people around you, that you don't hate.

Something that's easy to love.

Every day, take some kind of action to give love to that thing.

Eventually, when you're ready, try another part.

Maybe a part of you. A less-lovable, more scruffy part of you.

When you get stuck on this — and you probably will, once you get to scruffier and mangier parts of yourself — go back to the kitten.

In other words, give yourself a break by giving love, compassion and attention to something that's *easy* to love, feel compassion towards, and attend to.

This may sound cuckoo. But it's just basic neuroscience. It's brain training.

Love is a *practice*.

Compassion is a *practice*.

Attention is a *practice*.

What we practice, we get better at.

When you practice anything, you don't start with the hardest stuff.

You don't hit the Formula 1 racing circuit on your first day of driving lessons.

Similarly, if you want to change how you feel about yourself, and the behaviours you do, start small and easy.

Find the equivalent of the cute kitten to love and care for, whether that's a part of you, or a part of someone else.

And let actions build from there.

What thing / part / person do you hate *less*?

Is there any thing, part of yourself, or person that makes you feel at least a little warm and fuzzy?

What if you imagine a much younger you, maybe age 3 or 4?

Or your own child? Or a pet? Or the cute squirrel you saw in the park?

Or two old people holding hands?

Write down anything you *don't* hate, and would find easy to love.

_____

_____

_____

_____

_____

OR, DOODLE SOMETHING THAT
MAKES YOU GO

AWWWWWWWW!
AND FEEL ALL MUSHY.

Feel some good feels
on purpose.

Every day, practice feeling love, compassion, and care for something.

I know, I know, this sounds like the most hippie bullshit imaginable.

But it's the only path.

Criticism doesn't work.

Being a dick doesn't work.

Rigid rules don't work.

Vowing to *change everything* tomorrow doesn't work.

Neuroscience research shows:

Compassion works.

Gratitude works.

Care for yourself works.

But only if you let it work. And only if you learn how to do it.

That means *you have to practice feeling good things*.

If you can't feel compassion for yourself right now, practice feeling it for someone or something else.

Go stare at a kitten for 5 minutes.

When do we get to the food and eating stuff?

Right now.

But I'm gonna be tricky with you.

I'm not going to give you any rules.

I'm going to tell you a few things that work, and why they work, and you're going to have to deal with the discomfort of not having rules.

Rules might be part of what got you here.

Either you like to have them, or you like to break them.

In any case, rules do no good.

Rules are things that *other people* give you, and you have to follow them. (Or break them.)

Instead, I'll give you *principles*.

Principles are things you have inside you.

Principles are your values, manifested.

Principles are your "core". Your integrity. Your deep, gravid sense of right-ness.

Principles are yours, and nobody else's. You own them.

And just like your adorable kitten, you get to take care of them.

Wait, why is there food stuff in here at all?

Remember all that stuff about living in an industrialized country in the 21st century?

Well it matters here too.

Unless we're part of Doctors Without Borders or some other humanitarian organization working in impoverished parts of the world (thank you for your service)...

We don't know what malnutrition looks like.

So we wouldn't recognize it when it happens.

When was the last time you saw pellagra? (Aka a niacin deficiency?)

Or beriberi? (Aka a thiamine deficiency?)

Or kwashiorkor? (Aka a protein deficiency?)

Like never, right?

OK here's the thing.

If you have a history of weird stuff with food and eating and dieting and over-exercising and compensating and orthorexia...

...you may actually have nutrient deficiencies that *may be making you even more fucked up*.

Nutrient deficiencies can make things worse.

If you have any mental, emotional, and / or physical health problems, nutrient deficiencies from dieting, controlling your food, over-exercising, compensating etc. will very likely *make them worse*.

You might be at the end of a long string of diet and exercise interventions feeling crappier than ever.

Which is ironic, because you might have tried some of these hoping to feel *better*.

Outside of whatever else you're dealing with, repeated diets and over-exercise *themselves* may have helped to *create and reinforce* the problem.

Because malnutrition (which, eventually, these things create) makes you feel like shit.

Importantly, I don't say this to blame you.

You didn't know this stuff.

How could you, unless you specialize in tropical medicine or post-surgical nutrition?

I say this to inform you.

Whatever you're feeling right now might also be partly because you're missing important stuff that your body needs.

Remember: It's not your fault.

Here are some of the health problems that nutrient deficiencies can create or make worse.

Circle the ones that look familiar.

anxiety & panic

depression

fatigue

brain fog

obsessive-compulsive thoughts

infertility

hormonal disruption

thyroid disease

chronic pain

skin problems

digestive upset

constipation

diarrhea

irritability and "short fuse"

anorexia

low energy

headaches

inflammation

poor immunity

edema (water retention)

bloating

lack of mojo

poor dental and mouth health

dry and brittle hair

brittle fingernails

insomnia

losing your period (if you're female)

OR, DOODLE HOW YOUR BODY
AND BRAIN FEEL RIGHt NOW.
PUt IN SOME LIGHtNING
BOLts to SHOW WHAt HURts.

This is good news.

At least, I think so.

Knowing that malnutrition and nutrient deficiencies *themselves* can make things worse can be a lightbulb moment.

It tells you that it's not all your fault.

Your body and brain might not be getting some of the important raw materials they need to feel sane, normal, and OK.

This also tells you that:

Correcting nutrient deficiencies might help you feel better, almost right away.

You might not be ready to take this step just yet.

But on the next few pages, I'll explain some basics of how you can get started with an anti-fuckedup nutritional plan, once it feels like a good time to do so.

Before we get to *what* to eat, though, I'll start with *how* to eat.

Step 1: Practice breathing.

I know, I know.

This sounds so dumb and basic. You're already flipping the page.

Wait! Come back!

This is science!

To change anything, you need to know how to regulate yourself.

This means **you need to know how to calm down when you want to freak out**.

You can do this anywhere, any time, by consciously controlling your breathing. This helps lower your heart rate.

When you're panic-breathing, and your heart rate is spiking, you can't think straight. You can't act wisely.

You're almost literally scared stupid.

Calmer breathing and lower heart rate tell your body that you are safe and OK.

You always have this tool of breathing with you, no matter what.

So practice that now. Do the lung-sandwich, blowing-out-a-big-balloon slow-exhale, then a natural inhale.

Do five of those. Then move on.

Step 2: Eat slowly.

Take a bite. Pause.

Take a bite. Pause.

If you're used to binge eating and rushing, slowing down will give your digestive system time to process things.

You'll be able to be present with the food, and truly enjoy it.

You'll also learn that you can eventually sense into and respect your hunger and fullness cues.

If you're a restrictor type, you might normally eat slowly, so other people don't notice you're eating less.

You can use the idea of "eat slowly" as a way to be present with the food, and learn to tolerate the discomfort of having it near you.

Either way, remember to use the lung-sandwich breathing we learned.

Bite. Breathe.

Bite. Breathe.

Bite. Breathe.

Step 3: Practice noticing.

No matter what you eat (or don't), or when, or where, or how much, get into the habit of *noticing*. Observing.

Get in the habit of scanning your body, like we talked about earlier.

Add to your bite-breathe sequence:

Bite. Breathe. Notice.

Bite. Breathe. Notice.

See if you can sense into what your body is feeling.

If sensing into your whole body is too much right now, try an important part, like your chest or face.

Or an easy part, like your nose.

Just practice sensing-in and noticing those physical cues, as often as possible.

Ideally, do this while you eat. But any other time is great too.

If you find anything that upsets or bothers you, go back to your Step 1 of breathing. Take a moment, exhale, and calm down.

Don't judge whatever you notice.

Stay present. Don't check out.

Step 4: Practice believing that you are worthy of proper nourishment.

Oh seriously KSD?

Like fucking really?

Can't you see my body is gross / disgusting / stupid / not to be trusted / a rampaging greasy mess of gluttony?

Yes really.

Would you starve a baby?

Would you tell a patient in the ICU that they're ugly and don't deserve food?

Would you feed your own child garbage? (I mean literal garbage... like oily rags or coffee grounds.)

What the fuck?! No! That's a shitty thing to even ask!!

Well there you go.

How are you different?

If you are alive, you are worth nourishing.

If you are alive, your body is doing some magical things to keep you that way, and deserves care and compassionate caretaking.

Of course, believing you are worthy of nourishment is a tall order.

That's why I say: **Practice it.**

Just like parallel parking or playing the mandolin, you're not going to get it right away.

Every time you make a choice related to your body, like:

whether to eat

whether to not eat

what to eat or not eat

whether to exercise

what type of exercise to do

whether to get some daily-life movement

why you want to eat, not-eat, or exercise

whether to take care of yourself in other ways, like showering, brushing your teeth, or getting a medical checkup

etc.

...practice saying to yourself:

"I want to make the wisest, sanest, and most compassionate and nourishing choice for me in this moment... *even if I'm not completely sure what that is right now.*"

NOURISHMENt BINGO!

COLOUR IN tHE SQUARES tHAt WILL tRULY FEED YOU.

A HUG	A NAP	SPINACH
AN APPLE	PRIMAL SCREAM	TIME TO YOURSELF
SUNSHINE	SOUL FOOD	WILD ???? CARD
A HOT BATH	THE BLUES	KALE JUICE HA HA JUST SEEING IF YOU'RE PAYING ATTENTION
TELLING THAT ASSHOLE WHERE HE CAN SHOVE IT	FIRST STRAWBERRY OF SUMMER	A FOOT RUB

Let's check in with how you're doing.

Jot down some notes and capture any thoughts you have on the next page.

Any resistance to anything so far?

If so, what?

Are you excited by or interested in anything so far?

If so, what?

How are you feeling?

What's your immediate response to each of these ideas?

Breathing?

_____

_____

Slowing down?

_____

_____

Noticing & observing?

_____

_____

Believing you're worthy of nourishing?

_____

_____

OK, now we're getting
to the food and exercise.

Buckle in, because this is where some folks like to get weird about stuff.

Always remember the big picture.

Don't get hung up on details like *Well you didn't talk about steamed clams* or *What about the 6th day of Ramadan* or *But I can't eat avocadoes* or *My knee hurts so I don't ski.*

Charlie Chaplin once said:

"Life is a tragedy when seen in close-up, but a comedy in long-shot."

In other words, the deeper you try to drill down into something and control all the fiddly bits, the less happy (and to be brutally honest, less fun) you're likely to be.

So, relax.

Unclench. Breathe. (Always.)

Stop squinching your face. Let all your sphincters hang loose.

Step back and look at the *Gestalt* — the big picture, the context, the whole shebang, the thousand-foot view or seven generations from now. That kind of thing.

Step 5: Get enough protein.

Protein helps our body make neurotransmitters — the chemicals that help our nervous system send messages.

If we don't get enough of these neurotransmitters, our brain wiring gets all messed up.

We can get sad, or anxious, or lethargic, or fearful, or compulsive, or stuck in "thought loops" like a movie clip that plays over and over.

Protein also helps most of our body's tissues recover.

If you're restricting protein purposely (perhaps because you think it's "unhealthy") or accidentally (perhaps because you're a vegan and haven't made protein a priority), you might not be making enough neurotransmitters to make happy chemicals or other important hormones.

Add at least a bit of protein to every meal.

I've given you a list of foods to try on the next page.

High-protein foods to try

Here's a list of foods that are high in protein. Other foods have *some* protein, but these have the most.

Circle the ones you're ready, willing, and able to eat right now, and think about how to add them to your daily menu.

Remember: Proteins are building blocks for your body... especially your happy chemicals.

chicken

turkey

duck / goose

beef

pork

goat

bison

elk, venison

lamb

eggs

fish

seafood (e.g. shrimp, scallops, mussels, crab, calamari)

cottage cheese

Greek yogurt

tofu

tempeh

beans & legumes

protein powder (e.g. whey, egg, vegetarian blends)

Too easy? Bored of the Western Anglo standards?

Then challenge yourself!

Here are some other high-protein foods I've eaten on my travels.

insects and insect larvae

frog

escargot (snail)

snake

alligator

kangaroo

ostrich & emu

whale (3 types)

reindeer & moose

puffin & pigeon

organ meats including liver, heart, tripe, brains & testicles

turkey and goose eggs

beaver (hey! grow up and stop laughing... *uh huh huh beaver*)

At some point, I'll get up north and try seal, or give turtle soup a go.

If you're a Midwestern Anglo, you might see some of the above as weird and gross.

If you grew up eating these, it's just another day at the kitchen.

WTF?! Are you saying I *have* to eat bugs and sheep schlong?

No, no. Relax.

I'm saying that protein is important, and that you have lots of options.

And, as you feel more sane and curious about eating, you might want to try things or explore world cuisines that you normally wouldn't.

(To be fair, though, toasted mealworms are quite delicious, sort of like Rice Krispies. Don't so much recommend beluga or puffin, though.)

Anyway...

Here are some fun facts about protein!

Some people think "too much" protein is "unhealthy". They are wrong.

Much like drinking 8 glasses of water a day or the idea that saying "Bloody Mary" 3 times into a mirror will summon the evil ghost of Mary Worth, it feels "truthy", but there's actually *no scientific evidence to support it*.

In fact, studies have shown that up to 4.4 grams per kilogram of body weight of protein per day is... just fine.

To put that in perspective, for an average-sized person that means basically going to one of those cowboy-themed restaurants where you can get a steak the size of a loaf of bread...

...and eating two or three of those a day.

Nobody is *ever going to do that*.

So you are perfectly safe from overdosing on demon protein. It's actually much more likely that you can kill yourself with drinking too much water.

A higher-protein diet does, however...

- Help you build and keep those nice dense bones, strong muscles, and springy connective tissues for life.

- Help your immune and hormonal systems stay juicy and jaunty, full of zest and mojo.

- Help you heal, repair, and rebuild.

- Help your nervous system make the chemicals that keep you happy, calm, and smart.

- Help you feel satisfied with your meals, like you did something productive with yourself.

- Helps you keep kicking ass into old age.

Win win win all around.

Step 6: Add colours and smells.

Colourful fruits and vegetables (like spinach, berries, and carrots) are loaded with vitamins, minerals, and phytonutrients (aka plant chemicals) that do so many amazing things in and for your body.

The same is true of plants that smell, like garlic, onions, fresh herbs, or spices.

Colours and scents are your clues to helpful, health-boosting nutrients.

Every time you eat something colourful or smelly, you're telling your body: *Here. Enjoy this blast of good nutrition.*

And your body is all like, *Holy crap! Vitamin C and magnesium and sulfur compounds and fibre whaaaat?!* and gets super stoked about life.

Then it can go about its business of keeping you healthy, strong, and hopefully immortal.

Eating colours and smells tells your body that you give a shit about keeping it in good running order.

It's an act of love.

(Before you send me angry mail, I am not hating on celery, or mushrooms, or iceberg lettuce. All edible plants can be our friends!)

Colourful and stinky stuff to try

Here's a sample list of some foods that are colourful and/or smelly. The pigments and scents let you know that these plants have some goodies for your body.

Circle the ones you're ready, willing, and able to eat right now, and think about how to add them to your daily menu. (Or come up with others you might like.)

Red

Tomatoes

Red peppers

Strawberries

Pomegranates

Watermelon

Red grapefruit

Red apples

Red grapes

Red radishes

Rhubarb

Pricky pear fruit

Radicchio

Orange / yellow

Oranges (duh)

Winter squash, pumpkin

Carrots

Peaches, apricots

Pineapple

Mango

Orange sweet potatoes

Orange cauliflower

Green

Leafy greens like spinach, kale, collards, Swiss chard, watercress, arugula, etc.

Broccoli

Rapini

Green peas

Snow and snap peas

Green beans

Brussels sprouts

Bok choy

Zucchini (courgette)

Kiwi fruit

Seaweed

Green pepper

Purple / blue

Purple cabbage

Purple kale

Eggplant

Plums

Blue grapes

Beets

Blueberries, blackberies, lingonberries, etc.

Smelly

Onions

Garlic

Fresh herbs like basil, dill, parsley, fresh ginger, etc.

Spices like cinnamon, turmeric, nutmeg, cloves, pepper, fennel, chili

Mustard

Step 7: Eat healthy fats.

If you're a restrictor type, this is maybe the point where you scream "Peace out KSD!"and hit the exit.

Many people are afraid of fat.

It's true that fat is energy-dense, which means a small amount of fat has a lot of fuel stored in it.

It's also true that **certain types of fats are very, very important for helping you be healthy, happy, and sane.**

Fat helps make the membrane of every cell in our body. It makes up much of our nervous system and brain. And it helps build many of our important hormones, such as our sex hormones testosterone and estrogen.

Healthy fats mean healthier brain and body.

The omega-3 fatty acids EPA and DHA, found in marine life like fish or even algae, are particularly crucial for your brain and for controlling inflammation.

Research shows that people who feel anxious, depressed, obsessive, and/or compelled to have messed-up eating habits often have lower amounts of these essential fats in their brains.

Healthy fats to try

Here's a sample list of some foods that are high in healthy fats.

Circle the ones you're ready, willing, and able to eat right now, and think about how to add them to your daily menu. (Or come up with others you might like.)

Fatty fish (salmon, mackerel, herring, etc.)

Egg yolks

Avocadoes

Olives & olive oil

Coconut & coconut oil

Nuts (almonds, walnuts, pecans, etc.)

Seeds (pumpkin seeds, hemp seeds, chia seeds, flax seeds, etc.)

Butter (YES!)

Dark chocolate

Honourable mention as healthy fat superstar

EPA / DHA oil from fish, krill, or algae

DOODLE YOUR IDEAL MEAL.

WHAt WILL GIVE YOU MAGIC POWERS AND HELP YOU FLY?

Step 8: Move well, move kindly.

I'm going to use the term "movement" here rather than "exercise", because "exercise" is such a loaded term.

Plus:

Our bodies do so much more than "exercise".

They carry, and haul, and drag.

They move over terrain, traversing mud and hills and snow and rocky bits and curbs and all manner of obstacles.

They pull things and people close to us, or push them away.

They jump and run and scuttle and scurry.

They bend and straighten.

They balance and counter-balance.

They crawl and squirm and roll and climb.

They try to keep us safe.

The better and more lovingly we do all of these, the better our magnificent machine will work.

Not all bodies can do everything equally well (or at all), but in their design, *bodies are meant to move*.

Think bigger than "exercise".

Expand your horizons. Here are some ways to move that are not "workouts" or even "exercise" necessarily, just fundamental movement patterns.

Circle the ones that you can do.

Star the ones that bring you joy, give you energy, and/or help you feel powerful.

jumping	tumbling	rolling
crawling	swinging	stomping
rocking	pulling	hanging
walking	traversing	signing
stretching	circling	twirling
dancing	throwing	hugging
carrying	surfing	standing up
dragging	balancing	swaying
punching	riding	squatting
trudging	catching	bending
pushing	grappling	curling up
kicking	running	grasping
swimming	playing	hopping

IF YOU COULD MOVE LIKE A SUPERHERO, WHAT WOULD THAT LOOK LIKE?

DOODLE YOUR MOST POWERFUL & ENERGETIC SELF.

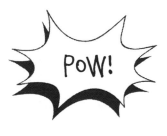

Somewhere along the way, we all got screwed up about movement.

We stopped seeing movement as a gift, something that most human beings have been blessed with.

We stopped seeing movement as a way of *thinking, exploring, problem-solving, and being in the world.*

Instead, we started to call movement "exercise"... or worse, "working out". We started seeing movement as something we do to "be good" or to fix / avoid "being "bad".

We started seeing movement as a chore. As discipline. As punishment. As inconvenient.

We fragmented our bodies into parts. We extracted our mind and consciousness completely from our flesh.

FUCK. THAT.

Movement is how YOU express YOU.

Movement is how you think, feel, perceive, and experience yourself as human. Emotions are just "blueprints for action".

If you could use movement to reveal your most authentic self, what might that look like?

If movement had *nothing to do* with "burning calories", "being good", or "getting abs / pecs / buns of steel"... would you do it?

Why or why not? And how?

_____

_____

_____

_____

_____

_____

_____

_____

Step 9: Repeat 1-8.

That's it. There's no magic.

There are no secrets.

There are only fundamental life practices that you must *do*, over and over and over.

Like *choosing* to slow down.

Like *choosing* to notice what is happening in your body and your life.

Like *choosing* to nourish yourself in all aspects.

Like *choosing* to behave with love and wisdom and compassion for yourself, even if you don't feel it 100% right now.

Like *choosing to choose*. Recognizing that how you act is a purposeful decision... *if you make it so*.

Take action. Action creates change.

Ask yourself how you can act kindly, right now, to alleviate your own suffering as much as possible.

Then practice.

Practice.

Practice.

And breathe.

Congratulations!
You made it.

Hooray!

You got all the way through this book.

Now the rest is up to you.

Change is not a one-shot deal. You're not "done" now.

Remember, you have to act, and keep acting. You have to practice, and keep practicing.

Nor are you ever "done".

Life is change.

Every moment is fresh.

You can start now... if you want.

Or don't. That's OK.

You're in the driver's seat now.

Welcome to the rest of your life...

...starting now.

Further reading & resources

Working with eating issues

Linda Craighead, *The Appetite Awareness Workbook: How to Listen to Your Body and Overcome Bingeing, Overeating, and Obsession with Food.*

James Greenblatt, *Answers to Anorexia* and *Answers to Binge Eating.*

Ken Goss, *The Compassionate-Mind Guide to Ending Overeating: Using Compassion-Focused Therapy to Overcome Bingeing and Disordered Eating.*

Karen Koenig, *The Food and Feelings Workbook: A Full Course Meal on Emotional Health.*

Sasha Loring, *Eating with Fierce Kindness: A Mindful and Compassionate Guide to Losing Weight.*

Geneen Roth:

- *Appetites: On the Search for True Nourishment*

- *When Food Is Love: Exploring the Relationship Between Eating and Intimacy*

- *Feeding the Hungry Heart: The Experience of Compulsive Eating*

Ruth Wolever and Beth Reardon, *The Mindful Diet: How to Transform Your Relationship with Food for Lasting Weight Loss and Vibrant Health.*

Change psychology

Barry Duncan, *What's Right With You: Debunking Dysfunction and Changing Your Life.*

Phil Stutz and Barry Michels, *The Tools: Transform Your Problems into Courage, Confidence, and Creativity.*

Self-compassion

Brene Brown, *The Gifts of Imperfection: Let Go of Who You Think You're Supposed to Be and Embrace Who You Are* and *I Thought It Was Just Me (But It Isn't).*

Kristin Neff, *Self-Compassion: The Proven Power of Being Kind to Yourself.*

Tami Simon, ed., *The Self-Acceptance Project: How to Be Kind and Compassionate Toward Yourself in Any Situation.*

Body wisdom

Peter Levine, *Healing Trauma: A Pioneering Program for Restoring the Wisdom of Your Body.*

Gabor Mate, *When the Body Says No: The Cost of Hidden Stress.*

Mary and Rick NurrieStearns. *Yoga for Emotional Trauma: Meditations and Practices for Healing Pain and Suffering.*

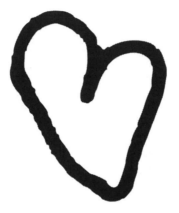

BE EXCELLENt to YOURSELF.

Made in the USA
Lexington, KY
22 December 2017